Large Print Short Stories

for Seniors

3 Books In 1

Felix Dalton

THIS COLLECTION INCLUDES THE FOLLOWING BOOKS:

Book 1: Uplifting Stories for Seniors

Book 2: Funny Stories for Seniors

Book 3: Interesting Stories for Seniors

Table of contents

Book 1:

Uplifting Stories For Seniors

Book 2:

Funny Stories for Seniors

Book 3:

Interesting Stories For Seniors

ACCESS THE AUDIOBOOK

Scan QR code to access
the audio version of the stories

— OR —

visit bit.ly/3FbqMzq

Introduction

The world seems to be moving faster than we can keep up with, and digital screens have become necessities. While technology has brought us closer together in different ways, it has also created a sense of isolation, especially among our beloved seniors.

But there is a timeless companion for generations that has always offered solace and even laughter, and that is the printed word.

In "Uplifting Stories for Seniors," we offer stories that remind us of the enduring power of the human spirit. "Funny Stories for Seniors" will evoke hearty chuckles and smiles, and "Interesting Stories for Seniors" will ignite curiosity in real and imaginary worlds.

As we go through the stories, let's remember that storytelling is more than an art; it is a bond that connects us across time and a bridge through generations.

Book 1:

Uplifting Stories For Seniors

1.We Owe It To Them

She colored the hollow letters a bright pink and tried her best not to cross the edges. "Happy Father's Day," said her coloring page.

"Mom, how does it look?" asked 3-year-old Zoe.

"Amazing!" answered Petty, who was on the couch next to her sister, Amanda, as she flipped the pages of her childhood photo album. The picture of their father hugging Amanda during her high school graduation reminded her of the look of pride he had in his eyes that day. The picture of him crying while walking Petty down the aisle reminded her of everything he's taught her to be who she is today as a person, wife, and mother!

"Are you going to color one for Grandpa too?" asked Zoe.

"I was just thinking the same!" answered Amanda.

"Maybe one that says "I love you" to mom too," added Petty. "We owe it to them," she continued.

2.The Drive-Thru Diner Mystery

"Hi, Walter" echoed repeatedly in the dining room of the nursing home, invoking Michael's curiosity. He looked around to see who Walter was. "No way!" said Michael.

Walter walked toward the buffet after greeting all of his friends and noticed a new set of eyes following his move. He stopped to see the newcomer. "No way!" he said. "Exactly!" Michael answered.

The old friends dissolved the lost years with a warm hug and a catch-up chat. They laughed at funny memories, showed each other pictures of children and grandchildren, and shared achievements and losses. And eventually had to bring it up...

"It wasn't you," said Walter

"Well, it definitely wasn't you! I'm sure of it," said Michael.

"She smiled at me!" Walter pointed at himself.

"And said, "Good to see you!" to me with a smile," Michael winked.

"Well, now we have a long time together to figure this puzzle out!" smiled Walter.

"Who did the cashier at the In-N-Out drive-thru like?" Michael held his chin and raised an eyebrow.

3.The Summer Camp Love Letter

He signed his name in the library registration book and headed to continue reading what used to be a trending novel during his teenage years, The Agony and the Ecstasy. As he picked the novel off the shelf, the image of the registration page flashed in his mind; her name was written right above his! The same handwriting even after around 60 years!

"Dear Johnny,

You're the nicest boy in our class. You make me feel all giggly inside. I'm raring to see you at summer camp.

Love

Samantha"

Johnny's always remembered the first love letter he'd ever received as a 10-year-old, as well as her eyes that he could recognize below time's gentle carvings on her face. He recognized her among 10 other visitors in the nursing home's library. He walked toward her table with the novel in his hand and said, "Hello, Samantha!"

She stared at him for a while until, slowly, her smile unfolded like a rosebud in the morning sun.

"Oh, my first love!" Samantha smiled.

"Mine too. You were the first spark that lit up my heart with love. Thank you," Johnny said as they exchanged a smile of gratitude.

4.Here Comes The Sun

"More! More!" a 4-year-old yelled at his twin sister as she poured seawater from a small red bucket onto the sandcastle her brother attempted to build. Their mother enjoyed a sunbath on her sheet, and half a mile away from her, three girls played skipping rope on the right while singing rhymes in front of their mothers, who sipped white wine in paper cups while taking bites from shining red strawberries and watching an interesting game of beach volleyball between a group of six men in their late 30s.

Ruth entered the beach on her bicycle, stealing everyone's attention as she peddled her way until she stopped right by the water. She pushed the kickstand of her bicycle and lay down on the cold, wet sand. She spread her arms and legs a little as she breathed in when the cold outgoing tide crawled on her, and she breathed out as the tide returned to where it came from.

The scene behind her was released from its pause. But the waves never paused anyway; they muffled Ruth's voice as she sang to herself the latest song by The Beatles: "Here comes the sun, doo-doo-doo-doo. Here comes the sun, and I say, it's alright."

5.Light My Fire

She took her mini cassette and walked out the door of her house. Everywhere she turned, she saw sharp-tailored suits, dresses, and miniskirts. Big beehive hair, pompadours, and extravagant hats were really hard to miss. Even when she decided to count the street tiles, she got interrupted by stylish go-go boots, classic ballet flats, and lavish saddles. They looked too sophisticated to even walk on the streets.

Simple moccasins entered the shoe parade. Her sandals weren't alienating anymore. "Come on, baby, light my fire!"

Her eyelids couldn't resist rising like curious curtains to gaze at his earthy green bell-bottom linen pants and the mini-cassette in his hand. As he passed her, a lively breeze touched her skin as she saw the back of his vibrant yellow tie-dye cotton t-shirt. His untouched hair sealed his mysterious face.

She looked at her red maxi skirt and smiled. She whirled gracefully, forcing her skirt to twirl and her bell sleeves to bloat like two happy balloons.

She pressed the play button on her mini cassette player and started to skip playfully, enjoying the walk and the song: "Come on, baby, light my fire!"

6.A Real Marshmallow Tree!

The crackling of the campfire, the dark sky full of stars, and the sweet scent of marshmallows filled the air.

Charles lifted the steel marshmallow roaster off the fire, and he and his 12-year-old grandson ate a piece in one bite. "Marshmallows back in the 60s were much softer and fluffier," said Charles.

Charles headed to a tree and surveyed it until he finally grabbed a branch.

"This is how you make a real marshmallow tree. You find a strong branch with multiple underbranches, strong enough to carry a marshmallow." Charles explained as he showed Jamie how close to the fire he should hold the branch.

"This is relaxing!" said Jamie as he watched white slowly turn to perfect gold.

As the evening grew darker, Charles and Jamie lay down to stargaze. Charles pointed to a constellation in the sky. "See that one, Jamie? Your Grandma used to call it the Nancy constellation. I've always seen it clearly from this spot, like a portal of a timeless connection between us and the universe."

7.What A Journey

With laughter and nostalgia, the old campers reunited, recalling the summers that shaped their lives.

"Do you remember what you said on your first hike with us?" David asked John.

He was only 25 back then; he's now 78. But how could he forget the warmth of the campfire that melted his heart and the orange glow of the fire sparks that burned his clingy attachments?

"This is what I want to do in my 70s. I want to gaze into the flames, relax by the fire, look back at my life, and say, 'What a journey!'" 78 John repeated what his young self once said.

Nods of agreement echoed louder than words through the night. In the crackling firelight, they found solace, knowing that their camp memories would forever be a cherished chapter in their remarkable journeys.

"Well, you've made it, my friend," said David with a smile.

8.The Soda Shop Crush

Suzie and Mark leaned on the counter of the soda shop, reminiscing. Suzie's long, chestnut hair cascaded over her tie-dye t-shirt. Mark's bell-bottoms brushed the linoleum floor as he ran a hand through his shaggy hair.

"Remember your first love?" Suzie laughed. "Oh! Billy!"

Mark's smile lit up his scruffy beard. "When you saw him enter the shop, your hands started shaking until you spilled soda all over Mrs. Henderson."

They chuckled, recalling the frothy disaster. "Uh, the 70s! The 80s should be fun!" said Suzie.

"Yes! It's the 70s mistake!" joked Mark as he sipped from his soda.

Mary entered in a simple white dress and green sandals. The closer she walked toward the counter, the less he felt his hand. He didn't leave his trance until the soda splashed all over the floor.

"You're right. It's not the '70s mistake!" Suzie teased him.

9.A Final Spin On the Airwaves

She pulled the brakes on her yellow Volkswagen Beetle when she heard the radio host present William Davis for a last Spin on the airwaves. As he started playing his DJ music, memories started to flashback; the first time she'd ever heard him, house parties, prom, disco nights, lovers, and even criticism from her mom, who never understood this new type of music. Tears of nostalgia flowed down her cheeks.

"Thank you for being a part of this unforgettable journey," William Davis said. "Please remember that every ending is the start of a whole new journey. So, enjoy the ride!"

With those uplifting words, the DJ signed off, leaving behind a trail of melodies that would continue to inspire his fans through time.

She started the car again and started driving.

10.   The High School Sock Hop Reunion

Neon lights ignited a sock hop high school reunion. Barefoot dancers floated as their hips swayed from side to side on "Rock Around the Clock" beats, capturing the era's groove.

Ladies twirled in poodle skirts while the fabric lifted as they spun. The gentlemen showcased quick footwork and hip swivels while donning leather jackets and slicked-back hair. Jitterbuggers spun and flipped, leaching out energy and excitement.

Circle dances told tales of unity, friendship, and love. While slow music brought bodies closer to each other, telling old love stories or starting new ones.

The sock hop dance embodied carefree, cheerful youth; that dance and music were the heartbeat of their generation.

11.   The Virtual World Explorer

Sam wore his Virtual Reality headset and started banging his arms in the air. His knees bounced, and his whole body was dancing.
"What are you doing?" Patricia asked.

Sam paused his game and asked his grandma about her favorite song. He handed her the headset, but she hesitated to put it on. She eventually did, after Sam's multiple attempts at convincing her. The big neon blocks coming at her scared her. She took a few steps back and took the headset off.

"There's nothing here, trust me! Just slash those neon blocks and enjoy the music!" said Sam. Patricia started slashing the blocks to the vibrant song "Somebody To Love." Each slash sounded like a drumbeat.

"It's like I'm a drummer!" Patricia was excited as she "played" her favorite song and bounced to it as Sam did. Sam started to bounce next to his Grandma, as he was happy to see her happy.

12.   Radio Hour

"Good evening, ladies and gentlemen, and welcome to 'Your Hit Parade'!" said Snooky Lanson through the radio.

Kenneth listened to the show with his neighbor, Donna. Each was in their room, but they communicated with hand gestures and smiles through their open windows.

"Listeners, we want to hear from you after this week's hit! If you'd like to dedicate a song to someone, give us a call. Our operators are standing by to take your requests!" said Snooky.

Kenneth picked up the phone and smiled at Donna, who smiled back as she watched him from her window, giving his request as Yakety Yak was airing.
"Welcome back, dear listeners. We have a special request from Kenneth. Kenneth dedicates this song to the beautiful lady with whom he listens to our show every Saturday."

When the music started, Donna smiled as she realized his romantic intentions, while he couldn't take his eyes off of her as his song played 'I Love You, Baby' by Paul Anka.

13.   Atari Is For Dads!

Jim, in his 40s, put on his plaid shirt and grabbed two chilled Budweisers from his refrigerator to join his neighbor, Mike, on his porch for a kickback session. However, he didn't find Mike in their usual relaxing spot after work. Jim decided to sneak a peek from the window into Mike's house.

"Don't you dare!" said Jim when he saw Mike keeping his kids' Atari in the entertainment center's drawer.
"They haven't been studying, brother!" said Mike.

Jim entered, handed Mark the two chilled beers, and set up the Atari set.
"Prepare to get schooled, my friend," said Jim as he handed Mark a joystick.

Mark and Jim started playing like their early 20s, in the late 1970s, were yesterday.
"Toast!" shouted Mark after he won!
"This version of Atari is 'totally rad', as kids these days say!" Jim added. They shared a good laugh before Mark had to keep it in the entertainment center.

14.   The Record Store Bromance

His fingertips traced album covers like a painter's brush. Thomas, a music-passionate teenager, flipped through the vinyl. He held Bowie's Lodger in one hand and Joy Division's Unknown Pleasures in another. A stranger's hand picked up Bowie's Lodger.

"Nice choice!" Thomas said.

"Thanks! I see you're on the fence," said the stranger.

"Yeah! I can only buy one album a month. So…" said Thomas.

"Me too! And I love Joy Division!" he shrugged his shoulders.

Thomas sighed as he looked back at the albums in his hands. He looked back at Bowie's album in the stranger's hand, then at Joy Division's in his. He put Bowie's album back in its place while making eye contact with the stranger.

"Great idea! I'm Joey, by the way," he said as they shook hands and made a deal to exchange records the next day at the store!

15. The Drive-In Movie Night

Under a starlit sky, cars lined up to offer a safe and comfortable haven for lovers. The big silver screen flickered as the most romantic movie of the 1990s screened.

While all the lovers were inside their cars, James spread a soft blanket on top of his car and shared a pillow with his girlfriend, Sarah.

"I'm flying, Jack!" said Kate Winslet as Rose.
Sarah stood on the car's roof, spread her arms, and screamed, "I'm flying, James!"
James burst into laughter before he stood behind her, held her waist, and sang, "Come Josephine in my flying machine. Going up, she goes, up she goes."

Soon enough, the drive-in theater turned into lovers on top of their cars singing, "Come Josephine in my flying machine. Going up, she goes, up she goes."

16. Whispers of the Twirling Skirt

Her fingertips conducted an invisible orchestra as she extended and curled them with every note of her favorite song on her mini cassette.

A radiant smile was printed on her lips while she shut her eyes to transfer herself to a different universe.

Her feet seemed to have a mind of their own as they tapped and pivoted effortlessly. She hovered, defying gravity, while she moved across the sandy beach.

Her hips swayed sensuously like a pendulum of rhythm and emotion. The stronger she pushed her hips and twirled, the higher her silky hair flew above her head, painting with its ends a painting of freedom that only dance can express.

17. Take It Easy

When I stepped a foot out of the airport into the streets, I heard a bell ringing in a happy melody and a voice calling in a different language that had a different rhythm to it. The mix of sounds turned my head toward it.

On my eyes' journey to find these sounds, I saw festive colors; red costumes, green accessories, blue sandals, yellow headwear, or a mix and match of all of that together. My eyes were overwhelmingly open to grasp the sense of fashion people wore while going to work.

He finally passed in front of me; an old man peddling on a bicycle, selling watermelon from a basket while ringing his bicycle bell and singing for watermelon.

A profound epiphany rushed all over me. I had a whole world in my head, but it was just a tiny dot in the midst of countless others.

18.   I Did A Good Job

Her son and his wife cheered while they were half submerged in the pool, encouraging their son to jump fiercely. A tiny amount of water splashed above the surface of the water when the 3-year-old boy jumped.

Her daughter and her husband ran around the pool, shouting, "Don't catch me!" while their 4-year-old daughter ran after them.

"Nana! Look how fast I am!" the little girl shouted when she got hold of her dad.

"Good job, sweetie," said Grandma.

"I did a good job, too!" she reassured herself with a smile.

Afterward, she leaned back against her chair, sipped from her chilled sparkling water, and put her sunglasses on. She enjoyed a sunbath by the pool and the sound of her family enjoying their time.

19.   Double The Chances

She mailed all the correct answers to last week's competition on the radio immediately and prayed every morning and night to win the grand prize; two tickets to Elvis Presley's concert. She already washed her favorite dress, ironed it, and hung it in her closet. She even shined her shoes.

She eagerly stood by the radio when she heard the host say, "Welcome, ladies and gentlemen," excited and terrified at the same time to hear the results. After an hour of listening to all the hit songs of this week, the host finally announced the name.

"And the winner of the two tickets for Elvis Presley's concert is... Mr. Frank..."
A disappointed frown formed on her face,
"Shapero! Congratulations, Mr. Frank Shapero. Your two tickets will be mailed to the same address you mailed your answers from."
"Dad!" she looked surprisingly at her dad
"I had to double our chances, my love!" her father smiled.

20.   Little Ball Of Fur

A tiny kitten wandered the street silently and alone every day. Her head stretched toward the ground as if she were trying to count the dust. Emily, a sweet-hearted lady in her 60s, saw her from her window and felt for her. Emily resisted her burning desire to take the little ball of fur home. She thought of all the grooming, cleaning the litter box, and all the bending down to pick up the little one when she would misbehave as kittens do.

Days turned into weeks, and the little kitten's neck stretched further down toward the floor. Emily had to give up one day and scoop the kitten up and into her warm home.

Days turned into weeks, weeks turned into years, the little kitten turned into Emma, the loudest meow in the neighborhood, and Emily turned into the most joyful grandma in the neighborhood.

21. Breaking Down Walls with Music

The drums kicked in, followed by the melodic guitar. Soon enough, the full orchestra had a musical conversation that David heard through his son's headphones. He glanced at Antoine, who spread an arm out of his window.

"I'm alone; yeah, I don't know if I can face the night." Steven Tyler's voice came out of Antonie's headphones.

David pressed his lips together as he looked back at the road's bumps and turns.

"Let's break the walls between us," Antonie looked at his dad, who started singing calmly, "Don't make it tough, I'll put away my pride."

Antonio settled into his seat and unplugged his headphones. Steven Tyler's voice filled the car.
David looked at Antonie and started singing: "Baby, you're my angel."

Antonie smiled at his dad and replied: "Come and save me tonight,"

The father and son duo blended effortlessly with Steven Tyler's voice, melting the rebellious iceberg between David and his teenage son.

22. Canvas of Forgotten Dreams

On December 18, 1957, Daniel, a dedicated art dealer, settled into his seat on the bustling train to New York. His eyes locked onto a seemingly forgotten canvas that leaned against the seat—a dusty and hopeless canvas. Intrigued, he examined the lost masterpiece.

It was a vivid depiction of urban life, covering a background of vibrant hues of red and orange dancing across the canvas, melding into a fiery blaze.

His long experience assured him that the painting was new.
"Mary, December 16, 1957."

"Good afternoon," the conductor greeted Daniel. With a great smile of hope, Daniel greeted the conductor, who seemed to have fallen from the sky.

23. Layers of Culinary Bliss

The man's taste buds ignited as he bit into the bakery's flaky croissant. Butter melted into its layers, harmonizing a symphony of flavors. His eyes closed as he savored the buttery, golden sensation. He chewed slowly and let the bakery's craftsmanship take over his senses.

With bated breath, Tom, the owner of the bakery, stood and watched as the critic savored each bite.

"Thank you," the critic said before he got up and left without saying another single word!

Days felt like years until the review was finally published. "A hidden gem, a testament to devotion." The bakery's popularity skyrocketed, yet its core remained untouched—a place where passion transformed into sweet success to prove that dreams could rise from the humblest ovens.

24. Reunion At The Eiffel

Beneath the majestic iron lattice of Paris, The Eiffel Tower, a curious set of eyes looked up as she strolled around the tower. The Parisian grace captured her attention, waking her on a timeless trip of observing elegance.

Stumbling on her steps, she returned to reality and into another trip, observing the faces around the tower; flirty faces, happy ones, naive, talkative, curious like hers, and even a familiar face!

Her curiosity couldn't stop her from staring at the Frenchman, wondering who he reminded her of. His eyes locked with hers, forcing her to send her gaze up at the tower immediately.

"Sarah!" she heard a voice say, "it's Chris!"
Decades apart, the Eiffel Tower witnessed the reunion of Sarah and her long-lost childhood pal from the States.
"I knew you looked familiar!" she said as the years melted away in the heart of Paris.

25. Ninety and Fearless

On her 90th birthday, Agnes dared to defy gravity. She closed her eyes as she leaped from the plane. The wind rushed through her silver hair as the world stretched below. She dared to open her eyes and see her lifelong dream of skydiving come true.

For a brief, breathtaking moment, age vanished, sounds vanished, opinions, thoughts, and ideas vanished—everything was in complete silence.

The parachute opened, and she gently descended to cheers from family and friends. Agnes proved that dreams had no expiration date and that life's most thrilling adventures could be embraced at any age.

26. Passing the Torch

Mrs. Anderson expected heartfelt goodbyes from her coworkers and colleagues. However, the room was filled with familiar faces—former students who'd become doctors, lawyers, and artists. Tearfully, she was credited with their triumphs as they remembered her support.

Mrs. Anderson understood that the difference she had made in so many people's lives was her actual legacy. The reunion was a celebration of a teacher whose impact went well beyond the classroom amid tears and laughter.

Her retirement didn't mark an end but the continuation of her profound impact on generations who will always be appreciative of her advice, insight, and faith in their potential and pass it along.

27. Fishing Tales

Under a warm afternoon sun, friends gathered at the local fishing hole. Lines were cast, and stories flowed. Mike recounted his legendary battle with the "one that got away" while Christopher proudly displayed his trophy-sized bass.

They enjoyed the company, cooked their catches on the grill, and experienced the simple pleasure of being together as the sun set.

The fishing hole continued to be a holy space where friendships developed, and memories were pulled in with each throw of the line. Their relationships grew deeper with each story told, each fish caught, and each fish splashed back into the sea.

28. The Sunday Family Dinner

Generations gathered around the table for their favorite family dinner every Sunday. The aromas from my grandmother's family recipes flooded the room.

While the seasoned folks shared their insights, starting their stories with "Let me tell you about the time…" the younger ones chuckled and listened with curiosity.

It was more than just a meal; it was a loving and interpersonal tradition. As food was handed around, tales were told, and hearts were united, the space was filled with warmth and nostalgia. Sunday meals continued to symbolize the steadfastness of family over the years, serving as a weekly reminder that love, like their favorite dishes, only became finer with time.

29. Margaret's Gravity-Defying Journey

On her 70th birthday, Margaret decided to venture into a new art museum and explore modern art. Unaware of the marvelous world that awaited her.

When she entered the visual arts section, her eyes widened in astonishment. There it stood tall, The Gravity-Defying Tower. Layers upon layers, suspended as if by magic.

A lady in her late 20s stepped onto one of the tower's walkways! Margaret's feet drove her closer to the tower to embark on an exhilarating journey. She stepped onto the walkway as well, and the world shifted.
Her heart raced with each step, and her worries dissolved into the void below as she floated with the tower.

Descending to solid ground, Margaret's free spirit radiated in her smile!

30. Silver Waves

In the park, on the adjacent lawn, a group of friends in their 70s swayed like graceful willows in a Tai Chi session. Their slow and deliberate movements belied their age.

Water splashed on the surface of the park's pool as lively ladies engaged in water aerobics while their silver hair shined as it floated on the surface of the water. Laughter filled the air as they kicked and stretched.

And on the winding path, ladies and gentlemen strolled, chatting and laughing, proving that walking was more than an exercise but a joyful social activity.

Their collective spirit defied stereotypes about age as they embraced a vibrant, active life at any age.

Book 2:

Funny Stories for Seniors

31. The Wrong Artist

Laura glued Pat Boone's picture on a canvas and added dancing musical notes around it. The poster sparkled with majestic glitter and artistic flourishes on its edges. She rolled it carefully, dressed in her favorite short green dress, and went to wait in front of Beverly Wilshire with hundreds of Boone's Babes.

Hours later, the ladies started running toward the entrance of the hotel like eager shoppers on Black Friday. She could only see his arm picking up posters and signing autographs.

Laura scooched in until she found herself in front of his car. He stood on the other side of the car, waving at his fans. Luckily, the car's window was open, so she threw her poster through it.

As he turned to sit, she saw his face!
"Oh no!" she said.
It was Elvis Presley unfolding Pat Boone's poster in his car!

32. Search For Tomorrow

Ethel's pickles became the talk of the town. For decades, neighbors lined up at her door, eager to savor the tantalizing tang.

One day, she sat on the front lawn of her house, chatting with five of her neighbors. Her grandson, who was visiting, joined them. They laughed at how Betsy fooled her children into eating broccoli cookies!

"What about Grandma's pickles? She fooled the whole neighborhood!" James laughed. Ethel didn't find it funny, though!

"I knew there was more to it than cinnamon!" a neighbor said.
They all stared at her, eager to know the story!

"I was watching Search For Tomorrow as I cut the cucumber. James was a teenager at the time. He cleaned up and found all the cucumbers but none of the zucchini! As a joke, he decided not to tell me until weeks later, when we opened the jars!"

She smiled and said, "Who's laughing now?"

33. Tech Grandpa

Billy looked at the pink screen on his computer with wide eyes. Grandpa Harold swooped in and pressed a few buttons on the keyboard of the crashed computer.

"Grandpa! Please, don't do anything!" said Billy. He started to hit Escape excessively, but it was all in vain as messages popped up out of nowhere on the screen!

"Oh no!" said Billy before he looked down at his feet and walked away.

All of a sudden, Billy heard the window startup song! He lifted his head and looked at his computer.

"It's working! What did you do, Grandpa?"

Harold smiled and said, "That's top secret!"

34. Funny Jukebox

When Tim saw Sally in Betsy's diner, he decided it was his chance! He walked slowly toward her, and his heart seemed to drop 100 inches with each step.

"Hello, Sally!" he said with a crooked voice.
She stared at him for what felt like hours, until he finally spoke the words: "Will you go out with me?"

The jukebox started to play "Love Me Tender."

"No," Sally said.
The jukebox suddenly switched to "Can't Buy Me Love." The regulars couldn't stop laughing at the psychic jukebox.

When Betsy served Frank his burger, the jukebox chimed in with "Big Girls Don't Cry."

Thanks to a jukebox with a knack for comical music taste, Betsy's Diner became the town's most entertaining hotspot.

35. Buy One Elvis For One

"What a coincidence! Look, urgent gig, tonight, $2000," a lady said.

Carl, the librarian, was confused!

"A massive '50s-themed event, they're insisting on Elvis, you in?"

He understood that she mistook him for a well-known Elvis Presley impersonator. Panicked but intrigued, Carl donned a sparkly Elvis jumpsuit.

He took the stage and transformed into a hilariously serious Elvis, with shaky legs, lip curls, and all. The audience couldn't stop laughing.

As the night progressed, Carl's impersonation skills surprisingly improved. "Did you know I once met President Nixon?" Carl asked the audience, using his background!

When the real impersonator finally showed up, the audience insisted on a sing-off between the two "Elvises." Carl's bizarre but endearing performance won the day and got him $500 in tips to replace the $2000 for the real Elvis!

36. Gnome-Sized Pie

Lucy and Eddie are a friendly neighborhood detective duo, or at least, that's what they fancied as groupies of Agatha Christie in the 1950s. One sunny afternoon, the duo stood before Mrs. Johnson's garden, looking through magnifying glasses.

Just as they were about to conclude their investigation, Mrs. Johnson's voice shook the porch. "What on earth are you two doing with my garden gnome?"

Eddie fixed his hat and said, "This gnome caper's the bee's knees, Mrs. Johnson! We're about to dust for fingerprints!"

Lucy nodded, pulling out a tiny brush to dust the gnome. "What's this gnome's motive to stay in your garden?"

Mrs. Johnson chuckled heartily. "Well, if you can figure out why he's been moonlighting as a garden decoration instead of traveling the world as a gnome spy, I'll bake you a gnome-sized pie!"

37. The Mashed-Potatoes

Amid a Sunday family dinner, chatter and nostalgia buzzed the gathering. Grandpa Joe usually embodies wisdom, but that Sunday, he revealed a hidden talent.

With a sly smile, he cleared the floor, dropped into stunning breakdancing moves, and grooved like a pro.

The beat of 1950s music pumped through the atmosphere of the 2020s. Grandma Edna couldn't resist and joined him, showcasing her funky dance skills.

Young jaws dropped as they started to drop some Mashed-Potatoes, Jitterbug, and Twist. A surprise turned into a thrilling dance-off where both grandparents and grandkids wowed the family, mixing dance styles to cheers and laughter.

38. The Gigantic Pie

A little, picturesque town had its annual pie-baking contest in the early 1950s, but this year was special. Competitors showed up with outrageously large pie pans that dwarfed their bakers.

Five workers held a slice of pie over their shoulders to serve the judges. Rock-crunchy crumbs fell and got stuck to the gooey butter that had already rained on workers' faces! Pies fell, competitors tripped over feelings, and laughter echoed throughout the area.

Tasting the pies was a struggle of its own; judges' forks hardly penetrated the thick crusts.

In the end, the winner was declared—the town itself, drenched in laughter and joy. The gigantic pie-baking contest had become a memorable occasion, reminding everyone that the absurdity of life can bring the most delight.

39. Pisa Burger

friends gathered for a meal in their regular 1950s diner, unaware of the new hilarity on the weekend's menu: "Biggest Burger Challenge."

The retro-dressed group enjoyed rock 'n' roll on the jukebox before the mammoth burger arrived. A huge and wobbly Pisa burger arrived.

Using extra-large napkins as bibs, one friend tried to fit the burger in his mouth, causing a cascade of toppings to rain down. Another made a makeshift burger barrier from hilariously oversized sunglasses.

The fries turned into flying missiles in a spontaneous food war, and ketchup bottles spewed sauce like party poppers.

Diners and staff laughed together while the cook came from the kitchen holding a giant spatula, pretending to flip the burger tower.

Although the "Biggest Burger Challenge" defeated them all, the group won a mess of giggles and good memories.

40. Town's Riotous Dance

The Swingin' Dance Contest took center stage and electrified the town. Couples danced to the upbeat music in the traditional swing style to open the event.

Later, a group of hip youngsters busted out wild disco moves, with flashy sequined outfits and exaggerated spins.

Next up, an older couple grooved to twist and shout routine, followed by a breakdancing duo who brought the house down with flips and spins that lifted the audience off their seats

Unexpectedly, the dance-off between a youthful breakdancer and a tap-dancing grandmother was the highlight. The audience applauded wildly throughout their amusing cross-generational duo.

After the contest, the entire town joined on the dance floor, the mayor moonwalked, and the postman busted a disco worm.

Just when the crowd thought they'd seen it all, the town's pet parrot escaped its cage and showcased its funky dance moves, flapping wings to the beat, leaving the audience in giggles.

41. Romantic English Assignment

Tim, a shy teenager, poured his heart into a love letter to his secret crush, Sarah, and kept it in his bag.

Days later, Ms. Sal read the English assignments. Tim's read:
"Dear Sarah, I hope you find this letter as thrilling as the mysteries of algebra confound me."

While Sarah blushed, loud laughter and chaos erupted in the class. Tim wished to crawl into a hole, and he understood that his love letter got mixed up with his schoolwork.

Soon, Tim found himself in the spotlight as the school's "romantic whiz." When Sarah approached Tim, his classmates started seeking his romantic advice, while others sent love letters inspired by his work.

42. Sunshine

In the groovy 1970s, free-spirited Sunshine stumbled into a high-paying corporate job. She dressed in tie-dye shirts and bell bottoms, and refused to conform to the sea of business suits and board meetings, Sunshine

She doodled peace signs and sprinkled flower petals on reports. Her every-meeting suggestion as a corporate strategy was "love and compassion."

Great chaos ruled one day as employees fought over chairs. Sunshine organized a "Circle of Love," demanding they close their eyes while she burned some incense and chanted: "Peace, Love, and Compassion!"

slowly, the employees started to cry, then burst into uncontrollable laughter while hugging each other tightly like a comical domino effect.

The corporate world never saw Sunshine coming, transforming the office into a groovy, flower-powered haven, showing that a touch of hippie spirit can work wonders even in the business world.

43. Rock Lobster

Alex poured his heart into a heartfelt mixtape for his secret crush, Jamie. The mixtape was a carefully curated collection of the latest love songs of the 1980s.

One fateful day, Alex nervously handed the mixtape to Jamie. She put the tape in her mini cassette and a bizarre mix of comical sound effects, strange noises, and quirky tunes of "Rock Lobster" by The B-52's.

Alex's prankster brother stood at the street corner, laughing while busting funny dance moves. Alex wanted to bury his face in the sand, but suddenly, Jamie started to bust even funnier moves!

Perplexed and amused, Jamie said: "This is the best love confession anyone could think of." Alex finally smiled and started dancing with her while stealing a glance at his brother, who was shocked the prank worked in Alex's favor after all!

44. The Cryptic Treasure Map

While a group of friends was taking a walk, they stumbled upon a memento of their childhood; an '80s treasure map full of clues that ignited their old, adventurous spirit.

The first clue, "Find the golden record," sent them scouring for vinyl albums. They found a golden vinyl with two songs, "Traffic Jam" and "Private Eyes". That led them to chase traffic signs. They remembered how the word "private" was misheard as "phone booth." They went to where they enjoyed lattes, a phone booth-themed cafe by a traffic sign.

"Head to the arcade" was their last clue. They were in a vintage arcade with classic games. At the Pac-Man machine, they found a real treasure: a stash of gold … tokens.

With joy in their hearts and gold tokens in hand, they spent the rest of the day reliving their 80s.

45. The Bill Buster

In the neon-soaked 1990s, young Timmy received his first cell phone bill, and his jaw hit the linoleum floor. It was so high that even the family goldfish gulped in disbelief.

Determined, Timmy made a business plan to tackle this technological monstrosity. He traded his sister's Beanie Babies for call minutes, convincing her that virtual pets were the future.

Timmy even began training pigeons to send telegrams instead of texts. He's also started his career as an organizer of the neighborhood talent show, all in an effort to pay off that monstrous bill.

In the end, Timmy's endeavors not only paid off the bill but also earned him a new title: "The 90s' Most Unconventional Bill Buster."

46. Jenkins' Kicks

In the 1990s, Mr. Jenkins, the owner of "Jenkins' Kicks," started selling sneakers with built-in voice-activated technology. The townsfolk, eager to embrace the trend, jumped on board, unaware of the consequences.

When debating the budget at a town meeting, the mayor's malfunctioning sneakers forced him to moonwalk. While the church choir's attempts to reach high notes during the Sunday service were blocked by the priest's sneakers, which confused "Hallelujah" for "Hokey Pokey,"

The school's librarian accidentally activated her sneakers while trying to shush noisy students. "Quiet, you hooligans!" her sneakers shouted.

Even the local police got some when he clumsily stumbled while shouting, "Stop in the name of the law!" at a thief.

The town's new wacky world of voice-activated sneakers became an unintentional comedy that had to be stopped in the name of the law!

47. Absurdly Luxurious

A group of friends decided to embark on an ambitious project: building the most luxurious treehouse ever. Armed with hammers, saws, and a wild imagination, they transformed a tree into a treetop mansion.

A glittering chandelier hung from a branch, a hot tub suspended from the branches, a treehouse-wide conveyor belt for snacks, and a mini treehouse within the treehouse for "privacy."

As they assembled the hot tub, water balloons fell from above, drenching them. The conveyor belt backfired, flinging sandwiches into the sky, prompting laughter and rescue efforts.

Neighbors were amazed as the treehouse got fancier, complete with a zipline. They rode it joyfully but crashed into the neighbor's hedge. The treehouse became a legendary symbol of friendship and laughter for years.

48. Beanie Babies Craze

Linda, an obsessive '90s Beanie Babies collector, auctioned off her massive stash online. The moment her listings went live, chaos ensued.

Her inbox was overflowing with strange inquiries from quirky buyers. One asked whether the Beanie Babies had attended any TV events, while another sought their astrological signs. A unique Princess Diana teddy went up for trade by one bidder.

With hundreds of bids, "Giggles the Giraffe" became the prized possession. The bidding war for the "Mint Condition Minty Mint Mints" tag protector erupted to Linda's amazement.

As the auction was ending, Linda discovered her dog had chewed up tags on half her Beanie Babies.

Linda's Beanie Baby auction turned into a comical series of mishaps as buyers acquired "rare" mangled-tag collectibles, and Linda laughed all the way to the bank.

49. Y2K Yikes

A group of friends huddled in their post-apocalypse bunker, stocked with canned goods and battery-operated gadgets. They wore aluminum foil hats and hung onto their goldfish as they counted down. As the clock struck midnight on New Year's Eve in 1999, the room became dark, and it was time to face the Y2K bug.

Time passed, but the planet held together. However, Michael's fingers were glued together from his attempt to seal the bunker door. And the fire alarm startled them when Tom tried to cook canned beans on the sterno stove.

As the night progressed, tension turned to laughter. The goldfish peacefully swam in its bowl. With the first rays of the new millennium, they emerged from their Y2K hiccup and bunker, victorious but covered in foil and glue.

50. The Walkman Woes

Mark was in a musical trance as he discovered the latest Walkman cassette player of the 1980s. He found out that he could record his voice on it!

As he bobbed his head to the beat in the library, the Walkman suddenly blasted out his off-key performance. Mark's horrified eyes widened. His cover of "I Will Survive" echoed, turning the calm library into a karaoke bar.

Library visitors started laughing uncontrollably. Anxious Mark struggled to silence the cassette as his cheeks became red. The damage had already been done, though, and even Ms. Shhh-annon Quietly cracked a smile.

Mark loosened up, joined in the laughter, and promised to keep his karaoke sessions far away from the library.

51. The Pet Rock Hoax

"Meet Zog, my pet rock," Terry said to his friends, gathering them under the steamy '70s sun in his backyard. He declared, unveiling a smooth stone painted with wobbly green antennas.

His friends exchanged skeptical glances, but Terry insisted, spinning a wild tale of Zog's antenna, describing that its messages could predict the future, from tonight's dinner to the winner of the upcoming NBA.

Some raised an eyebrow, but others were hooked. When the moment of truth arrived, Terry flipped a coin and "commanded" Zog to predict the toss. Everyone stared at Zog in tense silence. In a robotic voice, Zog miraculously predicted the toss correctly.

Panic! Friends begged Zog for answers, fearing the end of the world or their algebra test results. Terry finally burst into laughter, revealing a mini-cassette in his pocket and exposing the pet rock as a hoax.

52. The Destiny's Jest

Jenny, Mike, Sarah, and Kevin, four lifetime friends, laughed as they got ready to try out for a Destiny's Child tribute band while dressed in '90s style. It was intended to be a joke and a throwback to their adolescence.

However, something amazing occurred at the audition as they performed "Say My Name"—they were given the roles! They had changed into the phony Destiny's Child.

It didn't take long for the difficulties of playing the legendary girl trio to become clear. The Beyoncé impersonator Sarah tried to perform those well-known, energetic dancing moves but frequently fell over. Kevin struggled to keep up the sass of Destiny's Child.

Their debut performance was a flurry of costume changes, out-of-tune music, and mismatched dancing moves. However, it was well-received by the audience, who cheered and laughed aloud.

They may not have had the real Destiny's Child's swag, but they certainly had the most destiny-defying performance in town.

53. Friendly Radio Guy

The clumsy neighborhood delivery guy, Joe, stumbled into the radio station's control room as he was looking for who placed the order! He tripped over cables, knocking a stack of CDs onto the floor. The music abruptly cut off and panic set in.

He read the director's lips behind the glass window, mumbling: "We're live!"

He grabbed the nearest microphone.

"Uh, hello, folks! This is your...uh...friendly radio guy, Joe...coming at you live!" He looked around, sweat dripping on his forehead

Joe fumbled through the music library, pulling out random discs. "Here's... 'Wheels on the bus' by...um...The Driver!"

Oblivious Joe continued, "Now, a special shout-out to Mrs. Henderson's cat, Fluffy! Keep rocking, Fluffy!"

The host finally showed up behind the director, but they all liked what Joe was doing! Joe's charisma had unintentionally become the town's favorite hit with the audience.

54. Whiskers, Wigs, and Winks

The dimly lit basement of Mrs. Anderson's house buzzed with excitement as the ladies, dressed in men's suits, ties, and fake mustaches. They transformed into gentlemen of a secret club to whisk themselves away for a ladies night out in a '50s conservative town.

Tonight, they were off to the jazz club.

"Remember, ladies, we're the Whiskers, Wigs, and Winks," declared Mrs. Turner, adjusting her monocle.

Mrs. Johnson chimed in, "And don't forget our secret weapon." She held up a flask of "cough syrup."

They laughed, winked, and exchanged playful nods. Their husbands never suspected a thing.

Book 3:

Interesting Stories For Seniors

55. Time-Traveling Hendrix

With the intention of traveling back in time to the surreal 1960s, destiny sent Marty and Daisy to Woodstock in 1969 instead!

Amidst tie-dyes and tunes, they grooved in bell-bottoms and fringed vests. Marty strummed, and Daisy braided flowers. They joined a group of festival visitors who were exchanging "love and peace" stories and some "herbal refreshments".

A young musician by the name of Jimi Hendrix joined the group. They quickly hid their refreshments, afraid of churning up the history that Hendrix didn't even know about himself.

As Woodstock soared, they embraced the '60s spirit. No disruptions, just love. Their journey, unexpected but peaceful, added a colorful note to history.

56. The Disco Dilemma

Nostalgia drove a group of friends from the '60s squad to boldly infiltrate a late '70s disco soirée, donning their iconic bell-bottoms and psychedelic attire.

The DJ dropped some funky beats, but the gang started grooving with their flower-power moves, which were completely out of sync with funky DJ disco fever. They even tried to light up incense sticks on the dance floor.

When asked for their "digits," they held peace signs. Despite the puzzled stares and laughs, they soon became the life of the party, spreading '60s love in a '70s disco frenzy.

57. The Polyester Prankster

A mischievous '70s teenager planned a school prank by wearing a trove of hideous polyester clothes. He rocked those flashy duds, totally primed to be the biggest punchline.

When he walked into the school, weirdly, both teachers and students were in awe of his daring dress choice. Those disgusting polyester slacks and the garishly striped top suddenly became popular items. Soon, everyone aspired to have his bold style.

The prankster unwittingly became the leader of a fashion revolution after finding a vintage wardrobe in his attic.

58. Funky Time Capsule

A gang of groovy '70s kids buried their quirky artifacts from the era: lava lamps, disco records, pet rocks, and mood rings. They sealed them in a time capsule, promising to open it in the future.

Kids from the 1990s discovered the time capsule two decades later and were perplexed by the unusual artifacts. "What's this lava lamp thingy?" one asked. Mistaking the disco records for frisbees, they danced the "Macarena" with their pet rocks while wearing the mood rings.

Little did they know that these artifacts from the past would transport them on a nostalgic journey back to their parents' groovy era.

59. The VCR Voyage

Sarah and Mike, '80s teenagers, clutched their trusty VCR, their portal to the past, as they stared in disbelief at the unfamiliar room filled with CDs and a strange device called a computer. The weird sounds of grunge music echoed throughout the room, contrasting sharply with their '80s pop hits.

They struggled with the internet's alien technology, trying to find their way home, while their neon clothes and hair drew puzzled looks from those around them. Their only hope as they navigated the confusing world of the 1990s was to unravel the secrets of this decade and reverse the unintended journey through time.

60. The Retro Arcade Rumble

Mark and his friends challenged their rivals, led by Jake, to an epic showdown in the neon glow of '80s gaming center machines. The competition heated up as tokens clinked and joysticks strained.

The arcade games seemed to come to life just as the high scores were about to be settled. Pac-Man chased ghostly figures through the arcade while Donkey Kong threw barrels around. A pinball machine exploded in a flurry of lights and sound.

Laughter and shouts filled the arcade as everyone banded together to quell the pixelated rebellion, transforming the arcade into an unforgettable fun battleground.

61. The Superpowered Soda

A splash of cream soda spilled into the concoction as Benny, the bumbling soda jerk at the 1950s soda fountain, clumsily mixed syrups. Unknowingly to her, this mishap resulted in the creation of a new soda flavor that granted her temporary superpowers.

The word quickly spread, and the town was soon overrun with eager customers. People cracked up as they tried to control their newfound abilities.

With her supersonic notes, an aspiring opera singer shattered windows while a shy librarian accidentally turned invisible during a date. Benny's magical drink caused hilarious situations, transforming the once-quiet town into a bustling hub of super-powered shenanigans.

62. Rock 'n' Roll Reverie

Johnny, a teenager on the edge of adulthood, strummed his guitar in his garage in the heart of his small town, feeling the rhythm of change in the air. The sound reverberated throughout the neighborhood as the electric guitar's vibrant chords mixed with his voice. Johnny's soulful melodies sparked a musical revolution at the dawn of rock 'n' roll.

Friends soon gathered with instruments in hand to join the movement. The town square became their stage, and his songs reflected a generation's hopes and dreams. His coming-of-age story intertwined with the birth of a new era, forever altering the musical landscape of the great Johnny Cash's town.

63. Highway Harmony

The vintage car rumbled through countless highways under the broad skies of the 1950s, friends and laughter filling the air. They discovered the heart of America with each mile: roadside eateries with jukeboxes, neon-lit hotels, and pleasant people along the way.

They listened to Elvis Presley on the radio, marveled at massive roadside sights, and told stories around campfires under starry skies. The road trip became a remarkable journey through the soul of a nation, forming relationships that would last a lifetime and imprinting the spirit of 1950s America into their memory as they crossed state boundaries.

64. Red Scare Sleuth

The weight of a Cold War-era mystery pressed on Detective Malone as he walked through the calm streets of his little town. Whispers and anxiety spread among his neighbors, hinting at a decades-old crime. He dug through old files in the dimly lit archive room, uncovering a web of secrets.

Old images suggested unlawful gatherings, and mysterious phrases scrawled in code sent chills up his spine. The citizens of the town kept a close eye on him, worried that the truth might be revealed. Malone concluded that the only way to unravel the mystery was to navigate the delicate dance of secrecy and mistrust that had seized his neighborhood for years as he dug deeper.

65. Breaking the Mold

Susan, a strong lady with fire in her eyes, entered the bustling newsroom in the 1950s conformity. She wanted the opportunity to become a journalist, defying social standards.

As she challenged the current quo, the room fell silent. Undaunted by skepticism, she put pen to paper, writing stories that rang true. Her byline quickly made the main page, encouraging a new generation of female journalists.

Susan not only accomplished her dream career but also launched a revolution, shattering the gender barriers that had restricted women for far too long and blazing a route for change in a traditional era.

66. Channel Surfing Chronicles

The Smith family sat around the huge television set in their living room, amazed by the magic of the 1950s. They set out on a witty trip with rabbit ears antenna, and a flurry of black-and-white.

Dad twisted into ridiculous poses while attempting to adjust the reception. Mom messed with dials, making spectacle noises. Their children imitated the characters on the TV, turning the room into a slapstick circus.

They unwittingly captured the growing essence of entertainment through their laughter and blunders. The Smiths' early television days were a slapstick extravaganza in and of itself, a family comedy for the ages.

67. Soundtrack of Rebellion

David, a restless musician, strummed his guitar by the bonfire in the thick of the Woodstock haze. The counterculture movement whirled around him, a vortex of free spirits on a quest for self-discovery.

David's notes mixed with the heartbeat of a generation yearning for change as the music continued. He discovered himself in the glow of the festival lights, not in the glory he had sought, but in the harmony of like-minded souls.

Surrounded by peace signs and flower crowns, David's journey to self-discovery unfolded in the midst of a cultural revolution, a transforming trip in which the music was more than just a melody—it was the anthem of a generation discovering itself.

68. Summer of Love, Forever

Emily and Jack's love story unfolded in the heart of San Francisco's Summer of Love, amidst the kaleidoscope of colors and the strains of psychedelic music.

They met in a park filled with the aroma of incense. His tie-dye shirt complemented her flower crown. Their eyes locked as they danced to the beat of a tambourine, and the world slipped away.

They dreamed of a better future, a world of love and harmony, under the glow of a neon peace sign. In the free-spirited attitude of the 1960s, their love flourished, an eternal link woven into the tapestry of that amazing summer.

69. Cosmic Dreams

During the space race era, the hatch of the spacecraft opened, showing the lunar landscape below. Astronauts planted the American flag on the moon's lonely terrain. Millions of people stared in awe, yet in another universe, a science fiction scenario was unfolding.

In another universe, Earth's explorers had constructed a moon colony, which was a hive of human activity. Families flourished, and the universe became a playground for humanity. The historic moon landing marked the beginning of a new cosmic era, a monument to humanity's curiosity about the universe and the unlimited possibilities it offered.

70. Disco Fever Frenzy

The era's dancing competition began under the sparkling light of the shimmering disco ball. Participants danced to the hypnotic beats, unaware that their lives were about to take an unforeseen turn.

Samantha, a bashful librarian, let out her inner diva on the dance floor, gaining confidence that changed her life. Tony, a struggling artist, discovered his love for choreography and went on to have a great career. Even rivalries became lifelong friendships.

As the night progressed, dreams were born, lives were changed, and the spirit of liberation and self-expression of the disco period left an indelible impression on everyone in attendance, proving that sometimes all it takes is a dance to change the rhythm of your life.

71. Glam Rock Rising

In the vivid haze of the 1970s, four teens, Alex, Sophie, Mike, and Lisa, turned their garage jams into the rock band "Stardust." They took over the music scene with flashy outfits, electric guitars, and untamed hair.

They managed the era's glam and glitz, from wild parties on the Sunset Strip to sold-out performances at legendary venues. Their music, a blend of rock, glam, and disco, attracted fans all over the world. But celebrity brought its own set of difficulties—egos, and the never-ending desire for artistic expression.

They clung to their love of music throughout it all, establishing an unshakable friendship and making a lasting impression on the 1970s music scene.

72. Fueling Hope

The Anderson family's fortitude showed clearly in the middle of the 1970s oil crisis and economic turbulence. With gas shortages and rising prices, they abandoned their cars in favor of bicycles and public transportation. They tightened their belts at home, embracing frugality and ingenuity in their daily lives.

Once used to wealth, the youngsters understood the worth of a dollar. Due to work insecurity, the parents launched a tiny home company making handcrafted items. The Andersons' unshakable desire to weather the storm and support one another became a tribute to the power of family relationships, demonstrating that love and resourcefulness could transcend even the most difficult of circumstances.

73. Urban Echoes

A crime plot unfolded like a neon-lit puzzle in the gritty heart of 1970s New York City. Detective Mike Sullivan, a jaded detective, got himself tangled in a web of intrigue. Vincent "Vinnie" Marino, a flamboyant mob boss with a passion for silk suits and risk, was at its heart.

As Sullivan dug deeper, he came across a colorful ensemble of people, including Mona "The Nightingale" Moretti, a cabaret singer with a secret, and Jimmy "The Snake" Santoro, a crafty con artist. Twists and turns led to hidden agendas, betrayals, and a blood trail that covered the city's pavements.

Sullivan unearthed the truth amid the pandemonium, revealing the city's dark underbelly, where everyone had secrets and no one was genuinely innocent.

74. Retro Rhapsody

A bunch of misfit high school buddies embarked on a crazy coming-of-age trip in the vivid neon-infused pop culture of the 1980s. They walked the halls of adolescence with huge hair, leg warmers, and Walkmans in hand.

From big dance-offs in the gym to complex exam-passing schemes, their exploits were a mix of humor and passion. Zack, the school's resident heartthrob, became the target of devotion, while Lisa, the eccentric brainiac, devised inventive strategies.

This close-knit group discovered the genuine meaning of friendship, love, and self-discovery among the boomboxes and Rubik's Cubes, proving that even in the most colorful and wacky decade, the relationships of youth remained timeless.

75. Bits and Bleeps

Max, a computer nerd with a passion for video games and hacking, began an astonishing adventure through the early days of technology in the dark light of his computer screen. Max discovered hidden universes within video games as he improved his coding abilities—secret levels that stretched the boundaries of virtual reality.

But his exploits did not end there. Max discovered a mysterious online network of fellow hackers, each with their puzzling motive. They discovered government intrigues, digital treasure troves, and even an abandoned arcade full of buried riches.

Max's life evolved into a frenzy of unanticipated adventures and discoveries in the midst of bits and bleeps, indicating that in the realm of technology, the possibilities were as infinite as the sky.

76. Arcade Odyssey

A group of friends set out on an epic mission to uncover the legendary '80s arcade, which was supposed to have unique, mystical games long assumed to be lost to time. They crisscrossed the country with pixelated maps, following cryptic clues from old forums and ancient arcade cabinets.

Their adventure took them through neon-lit arcades, deserted stores, and underground gaming dens. Along the way, they encountered odd collectors, arcade ghosts, and arcade magicians who put their gaming talents to the test.

Their friendship was put to the test as they descended deeper into the realm of 8-bit legends, and they learned that the greatest treasure wasn't the games themselves but the shared experiences and bonds built on this epic journey through the golden age of gaming.

77. Cold War Craziness

In the midst of Cold War tensions, a satirical comedy with a cast of eccentric individuals entangled in international espionage played out.

Agent X, a fumbling secret agent with a love for disguises, became trapped in a bizarre web of assignments. Agent Y, an overconfident spy with an eye for electronics, was similarly useless. They went through a sequence of misfortunes including stolen blueprints, misidentified identities, and hilariously enormous spy equipment as a team.

The enigmatic Spy Mistress, a master of disguise and manipulation, tugged the strings in the middle of the chaos, arranging a comical dance of spies and double agents. As the world teetered on the edge of nuclear war, this amusing adventure through the world of spying demonstrated that sometimes, the best way to alleviate a crisis is through laughter.

78. Inventive Enigmas

A group of young detectives known as the "Mystery Makers" started on amazing adventures solving mysteries using their homemade gadgets and inventions in a beautiful '80s suburban neighborhood.

The crew handled anything from missing pets to neighborhood legends, led by the tech-savvy genius, Max, and his innovative companion, Lily. Max's radar-equipped bicycle led the way, while Lily's inventive contraptions, such as a robotic squirrel, supplied important clues.

They cracked codes, followed cryptic maps, and discovered buried mysteries with the help of their fearless leader, Sarah, and the tech-whiz, Jake. Each trip was an '80s-inspired thrill ride, proving that with a little innovation and a lot of friendship, they could solve any problem that arose.

79. Drive-In Romance:

Anne and John's love story developed under the starlit screen of their neighborhood drive-in movie theater in the 1950s. Every week, they'd load up the car with blankets and food and drive away to the wonderful world of movies.

As they watched movie after movie, they talked about their hopes and dreams, whispering about their future under the moonlight. Anne and John's love grew stronger against the backdrop of the era's challenges—racial tensions, societal conventions, and the ever-present terror of the Cold War.

As they confronted the complexity of the 1950s together, finding comfort and optimism in the simple pleasure of a drive-in movie date, their love story was a monument to the tenacity and the enduring power of love.

80. The Space Age Mystery

In the midst of the space race, a bunch of science-obsessed teenagers set out on an exciting adventure. Alex and Maya, inspired by the universe, unraveled enigmatic messages from space signals with their friends. Clues lead to the discovery of an alien artifact on Earth.

Their friendship became stronger as they traveled the world, deciphering old codes and discovering hidden chambers. Their trip was fueled by teenage curiosity and scientific enthusiasm. It showed that the wonders of the universe were within grasp, forming friendships and sparking a lifetime love of travel.

81. Culinary Chronicles

Betty, the spunky waitress in a small-town cafe, tossed witty banter along with orders. She supplied not only comfort food but also plenty of advice to the regulars. The grizzled cook, Old Bill, worked the grill with a continuous frown that concealed a golden heart.

The café was alive with laughter and chatter as the jukebox played '50s hits. Regulars shared stories, and newcomers sought refuge in the welcoming atmosphere. Love, laughter, and the ups and downs of life were on the menu, and in that restaurant, amid the scent of coffee and the clinking of silverware, the 1950s seemed like a simpler era of true connections.

82. Sock Hop Shenanigans

The high school's annual sock hop began under the shimmering disco ball, and the gymnasium was converted into a wacky farce. Students and instructors jived, parents whirled alongside teenagers, and mismatched couples danced with passion.

The principal moonwalked, a science teacher breakdanced, and the cleaning worker waltzed with the president of the PTA. The timeless appeal of the era permeated the gathering amid '50s music and wild dance routines.

Laughter resonated as generations linked through the enchantment of music and dance, indicating that the spirit of the 1950s was alive and well on the dance floor, even in the most unlikely pairings and joyful moments.

83. Bobby Sox and Baseball

Sarah broke gender norms with a relentless ambition to become a baseball player in the 1950s. Despite the skepticism and raised eyebrows, she practiced constantly, her glove and bat her closest companions.

Sarah's abilities surpassed those of the guys, and her enthusiasm for the sport was obvious. She established her worth at the neighborhood sandlot with each pitch and swing. Her ability not only inspired her community, but also defied societal preconceptions of the time.

As she rounded the bases, her dream and resilience demonstrated to everyone that talent had no gender limits and that the diamond was a place for everyone to shine.

84. The Hippie Commune

Jenny, a city dweller, sought serenity and enlightenment in a hippie commune set in the countryside during the 1960s. She imagined peaceful meditation and deep conversations about the universe. Instead, she was met with an unusual scene.

Hippies in flowing tie-dye robes chased butterflies, performed poetry to trees, and argued about the definition of the word "groovy" for hours. A goat donned a flower crown while a man played the didgeridoo for a bunch of chickens. Everyone looked to be high on "organic" herbs all the time.

Jenny couldn't stop laughing. In the middle of the craziness, she discovered a different kind of peace—laughter and a sense of belonging in the hilarious hippie commune.

85. Vintage Car Restoration

Dust danced in the beams of sunlight as retired mechanic Frank worked diligently on rebuilding his classic car in the dimly lit garage. The aroma of motor oil and the echoes of previous engines filled the air.

Every wrench turn, every chrome shine brought back memories of the open road—the wind in his hair, the purr of the engine, and infinite miles of adventure. Frank not only repaired the classic beauty but also recreated the spirit of his youth, recreating the delight of the open road one wrench turn at a time.

86. The Lemonade Stand

Young Timmy set up his kiosk at the corner of his neighborhood with a homemade sign and a jug of lemonade. His energy was contagious, and neighbors rushed to his sweet refreshment.

Timmy's tiny stand quickly became a bustling hub as word spread. His profits increased over the course of several weeks of hard effort, and the community rallied behind him. They noticed the young boy's passion and his desire to create a playground where children could freely play.

They raised enough money to make Timmy's fantasy a reality. The new playground became a symbol of neighborhood cooperation as well as the strength of a young boy's vision.

87. Words Unleashed

Emily, an aspiring author, eagerly attended free creative writing workshops at their tiny town's charming library. Her love of storytelling became stronger with each session, and her talents improved.

Emily wrote her first novel with the help of a skilled instructor and the encouragement of fellow writers. The welcome ambience of the library, packed with the aroma of old books and the steady buzz of creativity, became her haven.

She submitted her work to publishers, and her dream soon became a reality: her debut novel was published. Emily's transformation from a hopeful writer to a published novelist was a tribute to the power of community resources and the pursuit of one's literary goals.

88. Blossoms of Unity

Neighbors of all ages gathered on the once-forgotten lot in the heart of their neighborhood, equipped with shovels and smiles. They transformed the abandoned place into a lively communal garden with togetherness as their guiding philosophy.

Elderly hands shared their knowledge of caring for roses and daffodils, while children gasped at the wonder of growth. Tomatoes and cucumbers blossomed alongside sunflowers and zinnias, as friendships bloomed around them.

Their ties grew stronger as the garden grew. It became a haven of beauty and shared tales, with each bloom a monument to the strength of a community and the enduring beauty of collective endeavor.

89. The Heartbroken

Amelia, lonely and heartbroken, discovered a dusty jar of forgotten laughter on a dimly lit shelf in a world where emotions were physically collected and traded. The glass jar held brilliant, gleaming memories of joy long overlooked. She unscrewed the lid, releasing a burst of infectious and affectionate laughter around her.

Amelia couldn't help but smile as the laughter enveloped her. She realized that, amidst the rush of exchanging emotions, the simplest and most precious feelings, like laughter, had the power to mend even the loneliest of hearts.

90. Guardian of the Written Word

A hunter named Maya discovered a magnificent library unspoiled by time in a post-apocalyptic world where destruction ruled. Dusty bookcases housed forgotten information, their pages whispering old stories. Maya set out on a mission to save books from extinction.

Her lone companion was a ragged rucksack, which she filled with books, their weight a promise of hope in a desolate world. Maya believed these relics of a bygone past contained the secret to mending a world torn apart by anarchy. She would be the keeper of these tales, ensuring that knowledge would be passed down even in the darkest of times.

91. Harmony's Healing

A street singer named Jamie strummed their guitar with passionate enthusiasm in a noisy city area. Something spectacular happened as their fingers danced across the strings. The music had the ability to heal wounds, but only when it was performed with genuine care.

People passing by were lured to Jamie by the beautiful songs. A homeless man's injuries began to vanish, a child's tears turned to laughter, and sorrowful hearts sought peace. Jamie discovered they had a skill and decided to use it to convey compassion and healing in a society that desperately needed it, one meaningful note at a time.

92. Rescuing Tales from the Ruins

Elena, a lone scavenger, discovered a forgotten library among the ruins of a once-thriving city. The collected wisdom of generations was stored on dusty shelves. She made a solemn promise to safeguard knowledge from oblivion.

Elena clutched a treasured book to her bosom, knowing that in a world descending into turmoil, storytelling would serve as a link between the past and an uncertain future. She would ensure that the stories of humanity's achievements, tragedies, and hopes lived on, a beacon of hope despite the ruins.

93. Cosmic Direction

While stranded in space, John received cryptic alien signals. Symbols and patterns swirled over his console, strangely familiar yet mysterious. They became his lifeline, guiding his broken ship through space.

As the days passed, John began to wonder: Would these signals lead to his rescue, or were they leading him into the unknown? He followed the cosmic breadcrumbs, hoping to find the key to his salvation and perhaps a connection with a civilization from beyond the stars.

94. Bites of Memories

Each delicious pastry in a modest bakery tucked away on a quiet street carried more than simply flavor; it held stories, emotions, and long-forgotten memories.

Customers who bit into the baker's delicacies were transported back in time. An elderly man remembered his first love's smile while eating cherry pie. The aroma of freshly baked bread drove a woman to tears as she remembered her grandmother's comforting hug.

A sprinkling of nostalgia, a sprinkle of tears, and a dash of love were the baker's special ingredients, which were not found in recipes. Customers relieved moments they had long thought lost with each bite. Time stood still in that little bakery, and the past and present melded into a delicious, unforgettable melody.

95. Brush of Nightmares

The paintbrush moved with unnerving independence, turning the canvas into living nightmares. With each stroke, bizarre creatures and distorted landscapes were born. Desperation overwhelmed the artist, and he recognized the enormous work had to come to an end.

They clutched the possessed brush with shaky hands, their hearts hammering in horror. The bristles resisted, but determination drove them on. The brush fractured into fragments with one sharp snap, its sinister influence gone.

The artist gasped for breath as the pandemonium on the canvas paused, their sweat-soaked faces displaying a mix of relief and fear. The nightmare was over, but the frightening pictures lingered in their minds. They pledged that they would never again allow bad forces to rule their creativity.

96. Paws of Justice

An unlikely hero emerges from the midst of the animal kingdom in a future where animals have attained human-level intelligence. Whiskers, a once-normal tabby cat, took on the role of detective.

Detective Whiskers was confronted with a room full of suspects. He was keen to solve the riddle of the stolen tuna can, which had sparked a catfight.

As he examined the chamber of whiskered criminals, each one appeared to be more guilty than the previous. Paws twitched uneasily, tails flickered with distrust, and whiskers quivered with excitement.

Detective Whiskers realized he needed to rely on his instincts and sense of smell to solve the case. The stolen can of tuna had created a paw-sitively complicated dilemma, but he was determined to bring the feline society back to peace.

Detective Whiskers began his interrogation with a swish of his tail, aiming to unearth the truth concealed among the fuzzy suspects.

97. Echoes of Time

Dr. Eleanor Gray, a hermit genius, had invented a device that allowed her to rewind time in her solitude. The consequences, on the other hand, remained an area of concern.

Her invention, a tiny pocket watch filled with sophisticated gears and glittering crystals, had the power to change the course of history. But Dr. Gray was well aware that messing with time was risky.

She examined the options, the times she wished she could relive, and the lives she wished she could save. She paused, knowing that changing the past would cause unexpected ripples through history.

Dr. Gray locked her invention away with a sad heart, a reminder that while time could be rewound, what truly counted was the present and the decisions made in it. Time's echoes contained secrets.

98. Puzzling Chessboard

A chessboard emerged overnight in the center of the peaceful park, attracting the attention of curious visitors. Nobody knew what it was or what it was for, but one thing was certain: it begged to be played.

An unnamed opponent had already made the initial move, pushing a pawn forward. The question hung in the balance: checkmate or surrender?

Peter, a chess aficionado, couldn't help himself. He sat on the wooden seat across from the board, his gaze fixed on the pieces. He knew the game was more than just chess; it was a struggle of fate, a dance of destiny.

The pieces moved with purpose with each move, as though guided by an unseen hand. Minutes went into hours, and crowds gathered in wonder as the chessboard appeared to move and come alive.

Peter's heart raced as the final moves were made. But, in an unexpected turn of events, his opponent pulled off an unexpected move. Peter understood he was in checkmate after staring at the board in disbelief.

The invisible opponent, whoever they were, had triumphed. With a polite nod, Peter accepted the unpredictability of fate, where even defeat could include a valuable lesson about life's twists and turns—a reminder that destiny, like chess, was unpredictable and ever-changing.

99. Ground Control

Captain Sarah Mitchell, a trapped astronaut on Mars, had given up hope of ever returning home. Her foot kicked something beneath the red dust as she trekked over the dim landscape—a metal plate inscribed with the words "I Found Answers Here."

She followed a list of locations carved on the plate, intrigued and anxious for any indication of civilization. She uncovered a concealed box with a handwritten journal miles away. It was the log of a former visitor, whose identity was unknown.

Sarah perused the journal with increasing interest. It mentioned old Martian relics, strange events, and mysteries hidden beneath Martian soil. The author thought they had found solutions to fundamental puzzles regarding the universe.

Sarah set off on a fascinating adventure across the bleak countryside, guided by the enigmatic notes left behind. She was determined to discover the truth. As she dug more into the Martian puzzles, she realized that the solutions she sought were entwined with the planet's hidden history.

100. Thunderous Past

Emma Riley tracked storms in order to capture nature's fury. Her lens took a magnificent photograph of an electric lightning strike that lit up the sky like a celestial firework on a stormy night. But as she looked over the shot, she noticed something unusual—a hidden message.

Fascinating patterns and symbols developed within the lightning's jagged course. Emma couldn't believe what she was seeing. It was as if the lightning had imprinted a message from the past on the sensor of her camera.

Emma's interest motivated her to translate the symbols, which resembled ancient hieroglyphs. Days stretched into weeks, and she realized that the lightning carried a message from a long-gone civilization. It suggested the existence of a lost metropolis buried beneath the soil.

Determined to discover the truth, she had no idea that the snapshot she had taken would take her on an incredible journey into the depths of history and the mysteries of the past.

101. The Enchanted Carnival

A weird circus appeared on the outskirts of town one rainy evening. Curiosity drew the townspeople inside the gloomy tent, oblivious to the bizarre scene that awaited them.

Inside, the performances were unlike anything they'd ever seen before: acrobats with moonlight wings, jugglers who held fire with their bare hands, and a ringmaster with eyes that contained the secrets of the cosmos.

The crowd became a part of the surreal act as the night progressed. They float weightlessly, dance on air, and even communicate with ethereal beings. The divide between audience and actor dissolved as reality and fiction merged.

As daylight neared, though, the circus began to vanish, leaving the crowd in amazement and wonder. They returned to town with unforgettable recollections of a night transformed by the enchantment of the mysterious carnival.

102. The Forgotten Love Letters

Amelia discovered a hidden area behind a dusty bookcase while touring her grandmother's ancient house. She discovered a treasure trove of letters, each written with love and desire.

The letters revealed a long-dormant relationship between Eleanor, her grandma, and a hidden lover named Samuel. Amelia was attracted by their emotional writings, which recounted stolen glances, whispered pledges, and shared hopes for a future together.

Amelia set out on a journey through fading images, dusty journals, and yellowed letters to discover Samuel's identity. She put together the beautiful yet heartbreaking love tale of her grandmother's history with each revelation.

In the end, Amelia uncovered Samuel's actual identity and the barriers that had kept him and Eleanor apart. Though time had separated the lovers, Amelia's journey allowed her to bridge the distance and acknowledge the undying love that had previously bloomed within the hidden room.

103. The Librarian's Guardian

Librarian Lydia owned a cherished and irreversible secret in a world where books had the ability to influence destinies—a prohibited tome concealed deep behind the labyrinthine shelves of the Great Library.

The book held prophecies and information so powerful that its pure presence jeopardized the world's fragile balance. It had been kept secret for generations to avoid coming into the hands of the wrong people.

A wicked stranger entered the library one fateful day, his eyes burning with thirst for the forbidden information. Lydia, the tome's keeper, understood she had to defend it at all costs.

Lydia and the intruder danced between the racks of old scrolls in a cat-and-mouse quest through the dimly lighted halls. Finally, in a desperate move, Lydia unleashed the book's power, changing the intruder's motives and leaving them stunned by its potential for good.

Lydia, the book's dedicated guardian, continued to shield the future from the wrong hands, ensuring its pages never fell into darkness.

104. Chronicles of the Time Train

A sharp shock left people spreading as the commuter train barreled down the rails. When they recovered consciousness, they found themselves in a foreign terrain, having been transferred to a different time and location.

As they grasped their predicament, their confusion turned to terror. The interior of the train has been changed, with vintage furnishings replacing contemporary seats. Outside, the environment was similarly perplexing—a bygone past buzzing with horse-drawn vehicles and gas lamps.

Strangers became friends as they banded together to investigate the riddle of their relocation. They investigated a cryptic chart found in the conductor's cabin, gradually understanding the mystery of their journey.

They weathered the obstacles of this strange new environment together, forming relationships that would last a lifetime. Their only hope was to understand the chart and find their way back home, but they had no idea that this unexpected adventure would alter them and leave an everlasting stamp on each passenger's heart.

105. The Celestial Serenade

Struggling musician Oliver found a fascinating instrument unlike any other in the deepest reaches of an ancient music store—a dazzling, heavenly harp with strings that seemed to resonate with the heartbeat of the cosmos.

The room was filled with an amazing tune that exceeded the limitations of human imagination as he stroked the harp's strings. He had no idea that his music would be heard far beyond Earth's borders.

Celestial creatures descended from the sky, captivated by the ethereal harmonies, to watch the earthly musician who had unlocked the music of the stars. They danced in the moonlight, their glowing forms swirling about Oliver as they sang a magnificent symphony.

As he played with these unearthly entities, Oliver's heart flooded with wonder. The symphony of the cosmos had shown him the limitless beauty of the universe.

The celestial entities retreated to the heavens as morning came, leaving Oliver in wonder and knowing that the power of music could transcend the gap between the earthly and the holy.

106. Dreams for Sale

Daniel had developed a dangerous fixation in a society where dreams were commodities. He began by purchasing dreams of adventure, love, and faraway locations, experiencing the pleasure of living via the nocturnal voyages of others. However, as time progressed, the line between his actual reality and his dream world became increasingly blurred.

Daniel was obsessed with his passion every waking minute, accumulating dreams that didn't belong to him, their borders and repercussions slipping into oblivion. He developed an addiction to the excitement of experiencing countless lives in his sleep.

Daniel lost touch with reality as he descended deeper into this terrible addiction. He was caught in a labyrinth of stolen dreams, and his identity was shattered.

Daniel was jolted awake by a terrifying nightmare—his own dream. He recognized the price of his obsession had become his own life, dreams, and sanity. He had lost the most valuable fantasy of all—his own reality—in a world where fantasies were bought and dealt with.

107. The Midnight Escapade

A street artist called Mia created a mural in the center of the city that caught the spirit of urban life. Her creation, however, carried a secret: as night fell, the characters on the wall came to life, escaping the bounds of their painted world.

Mia's figures sprang off the wall one beautiful night while the city slept, led by a cheeky graffiti tagger. They strolled the dark streets, having their own adventures. The spray-can-wielding tagger created a colorful trail of art around the city.

Mia, a street artist, drew a painting in the city center that captured the energy of urban life. Her work, on the other hand, held a secret: once darkness fell, the characters on the wall sprang to life, breaking free from the confines of their painted world.

Mia's figures appeared on the wall one glorious night while the city slept, guided by a mischievous graffiti tagger. They were enjoying their own experiences as they went through the nighttime alleys. The spray-can-wielding tagger left a colorful trail of art all across town.

108. The Forgotten Pharaoh

Dr. Amelia Reynolds, a courageous archaeologist, had discovered many mysteries throughout her career, but nothing had prepared her for the tomb she discovered deep under the Egyptian desert. Inside, hieroglyphs warned of a terrible curse—a malignant entity trapped for millennia.

Amelia ignored the warnings and dug further, her interest overcoming her prudence. A peculiar sensation flooded over her as she neared the sarcophagus of the long-forgotten Pharaoh, and a chilling mumble resonated through the hall.

The curse had been awakened.

Amelia understood she was imprisoned as the tomb closed behind her. The curse's hold increased with each passing day, sapping her power and warping her reality. She had no option but to answer the ancient riddles that held the secret to releasing the curse.

Amelia's life was hanging in the balance as time ran short. She started on a perilous trek in the heart of the tomb to uncover the curse's mysteries and rescue herself from its terrible clutches before it destroyed her entirely.

109. A Glimpse Through Time

Ella, a single mother, worked the night shift at a quiet convenience store, hoping for a better life for herself and her kid. Her ordinary life took a bizarre turn one night.

She observed something strange while watching the security camera footage—the images on the screen moved, exposing moments from the past. She saw clients and their secrets, moments that had passed but were caught by the camera's unfathomable power.

Ella's heart beat faster as she caught sight of secret kisses, touching confessions, and whispered pledges. The webcam had become a doorway into her customers' private histories.

Ella became a mute witness to the pleasures and sorrows of strangers' lives throughout time. She found herself empathizing with their tales and connecting with them from afar. Her awareness of human nature grew, and she learned that extraordinary moments and secrets might be revealed even in the most ordinary of settings.

Ella kept her silent vigil throughout the night, feeling a newfound appreciation for the numerous untold stories that unfolded before her eyes.

110. The Parallel Paradox

Walter, a struggling inventor, labored in his chaotic studio for hours on end to construct a gadget that might solve the riddles of parallel worlds. When he eventually succeeded, he allowed individuals to see their other selves, each of whom was living a different life.

The gadget became an instant hit. People came to their parallel worlds to enjoy the endless possibilities. Walter basked in the happiness he had provided to others. However, as more individuals investigated, it became increasingly impossible for them to return to their own world.

They got engrossed in their parallel lives one by one, ignoring their obligations in the present. Walter stared in dismay as the boundary between reality and fantasy blurred.

Walter made a heartbreaking decision in order to prevent his invention from causing additional pain. He destroyed the apparatus, aware that the appeal of parallel universes was a two-edged sword.

In the end, the inventor's greatest creation became his greatest sacrifice, a warning that the quest for boundless possibilities may often result in the loss of the one reality that matters most.

111. The Parallel Paradox

Walter, a struggling inventor, labored in his chaotic studio for hours on end to construct a gadget that might solve the riddles of parallel worlds. When he eventually succeeded, he allowed individuals to see their other selves, each of whom was living a different life.

The gadget became an instant hit. People came to their parallel worlds to enjoy the endless possibilities. Walter basked in the happiness he had provided to others. However, as more individuals investigated, it became increasingly impossible for them to return to their own world.

They got engrossed in their parallel lives one by one, ignoring their obligations in the present. Walter stared in dismay as the boundary between reality and fantasy blurred.

Walter made a heartbreaking decision in order to prevent his invention from causing additional pain. He destroyed the apparatus, aware that the appeal of parallel universes was a two-edged sword.

In the end, the inventor's greatest creation became his greatest sacrifice, a warning that the quest for boundless possibilities may often result in the loss of the one reality that matters most.

112. The Beekeeper's Revelation

Emma, a beekeeper in the calm village of Willowbrook, discovered an inexplicable shift in her beloved bees. They danced in strange rhythms, making intricate forms in the air that went beyond normal bee communication.

Emma, with her strong connection to the hive, realized something important was taking place in front of her. She examined the bees for days, understanding their sophisticated choreography, determined to interpret this enigmatic message.

Emma began to detect a hidden message encoded into their dances as she studied them—a warning of an approaching environmental calamity that would endanger the village. The bees had detected the coming threat because they were tuned into the world's rhythms.

Emma jumped into action, informing the townspeople and preparing for the approaching disaster. She was fueled by the urgency of their message. The community of Willowbrook was able to unify and protect itself thanks to the bees' amazing communication, demonstrating that even the smallest animals may carry the knowledge to guide humans through the most difficult circumstances.

113. The Glasses of Truth

Alex, a teenager, came into a dusty pair of glasses concealed in the attic one routine day. When he put them on, the world altered before his eyes. The glasses exposed the genuine character of people's thoughts and intentions, which he found both amusing and depressing.

As he proceeded down the street, he noticed Mr. Johnson, whose pleasant appearance belied his yearning for his beloved rosebush. Sarah, his best friend at school, had a crush on him that she had never acknowledged. And Max, the class bully, was insecure and lonely.

Some disclosures were funny, while others were disturbing. People's latent preconceptions and biases were revealed, resulting in terrible disappointment. Knowing the unvarnished truth about people wasn't always a blessing; it came with the responsibility of comprehending the complexity of human nature.

With a sad heart, he removed his glasses, opting to traverse the world with understanding and compassion, knowing that the truth was often better left unsaid.

Conclusion

We've taken a journey through the pages of "Large Print Short Stories for Seniors" through laughter, tears, and wonder. As we near the end of this literary journey, it's crucial to consider the significant impact that stories have on our lives, particularly those of our beloved seniors.

The stories in this 3-book set have reminded us of the everlasting power of storytelling, whether they made us laugh out loud, aroused our interest, or pulled at our heartstrings. These stories have offered solace to many who may have felt alone in a world that is dominated by digital devices and rapid change. They have shown that the printed word could serve as a reliable companion in times of solitude.

As we finish the book on "Interesting Stories for Seniors," we are left with a profound respect for the persistence of the human spirit and the unifying power of storytelling. These stories have functioned as a link between generations, linking us to our elders' knowledge and the young's curiosity. They have demonstrated that, no matter how fast the world around us changes, the power of a well-told story can survive, providing solace, joy, and a timeless connection.

May we carry the warmth of these stories with us in the quiet moments after the last page is turned, and may they continue to uplift the hearts of seniors and readers of all ages, reminding us that the art of storytelling is a valuable gift that can enrich our lives and bind us together, no matter how fast the world appears to spin.